THAT'S S[...] FORGOT TO LAUGH

Facing a cancer recurrence
By:
Lauren Brower

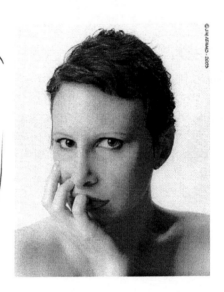

Bookman Publishing
Martinsville, Indiana
www.BookmanMarketing.com

*Best Wishes
Lauren Brower*

ISBN: 1-59453-055-6

Acknowledgements

I have to thank God for the gift of my family and friends who have supported me in many ways through my treatment, recovery and the process of sharing through writing and speaking. I give thanks to my husband Scott for being the patient man he promised to be so many years ago. I am grateful that I trusted him. I must thank my parents who are uniquely special and unlike any others on this earth. If there are earthbound people that are bound for heaven, my mother and father will be among that number. The late night phone calls, the constant visits, the laundry, the angry outbursts and the confused crying fits never stopped the overflowing love and all powerful hugs, not to mention the late night backrubs that can always calm the savage beast.

Of course I must thank my doctors for allowing me to be a person and not a patient. To Dr. Cloninger a second father, I love you dearly. To Dr. Mitchell whom I trust implicitly for my care and his musical taste, and Dr. Mogabgab for trusting his instincts and for caring so much.

I owe a debt of gratitude to my friends too many to mention, still I must try to address some of them. To Holly who makes such efforts to be strong and supportive. To Kim, who even from a distance never wants to leave my side. To Steve P and his lovely wife Morgan who always ask the magic question, "How are you?" I love you because you mean it. I would be remiss not to thank Brandi G. for her work with my first book. To the Richey family for support.

Thanks to all the musicians; Scott, Adrian, Rick, Marshall, Dave, Mike, Clayton, Louis, Mark, and Frank for covering for me when I was comatose and for making me look like a real diva even when I didn't look or sound like one.

To the Wine Vault for years of support and allowing me to sing on Morphine. Likewise thanks to the Village Tavern, Birkdale Village and our agents for continued support through the years as well. To the regulars who come to hear us over and over, and our new fans who quickly lend their support and to those who listen to me talk about this dread disease.

Hats off to the other fighters who have fought bravely before us and gone on. Thank you for your spirits.

Lauren
"The Diva"

Introduction

Cancer the second time around is a different beast. At least that has been my personal experience. During and after my original treatment for breast cancer in Oct. of 2000, I had a tremendous sense of hope and accomplishment. I was 34. I still felt young and strong and I was certain if I followed the regimen with the right attitude and devotion that I would beat this disease and have a new life. Indeed for 2 years I continued to be disease free and found a renewed sense of self. It permeated all that I touched. I was a changed woman.

Still, while the change was obvious, the path of my life was not so clear. I was so overwhelmed with options that I wanted to try everything, which of course led me to accomplish less than I had hoped. My days were almost normal again. The sales of the book I wrote on my experience (partly for my own therapy and partly to help others) dwindled, I didn't even mention it in general conversations as I had done previously. In fact the whole idea that I had even been treated for cancer seemed foreign. No one really brought it up anymore, and though I was still proud for beating it, and beating it so young, I had stopped making it part of my identity. Looking back I can see that I was killing myself by trying to "live life to the fullest". I felt I had to take on the world fearlessly and I tried to swallow the whole thing like a big pill. I should have realized living life meant taking time for reflection and renewal. That realization came quickly enough.

In the midst of my renaissance I felt a nagging in my chest. That isn't a figurative statement. In the period of a week or so I began to feel what felt like congestion from a cold. It hurt if I took a deep breath. A week later I sat in my General

Practitioner's office after hours. He called me there to tell me that a scan he ordered "just to be sure" is showing lesions in my sternum. I sat in shock. I hadn't won the war, only a battle. The cancer was back, and it was back in my bones.

I really didn't understand the implications of that at the moment. I didn't know that I was now classified as Stage IV and that technically my disease was "incurable". All I knew is that I had somehow failed. My body had failed. I was almost too overwhelmed to cry. That is until I got in the car and started heading home. The floodgates opened.

I searched hard to find the sense of humor I had always relied on, the one that I wrote that whole book about. I felt myself a hypocrite for advocating the power of laughter in healing so many times before. I feared I might not ever find it again. Eventually I realized that I didn't immediately discover the value of my sense of humor after my first diagnosis until well into treatment, and almost by accident. So why would I think this time would be so different? I came to a fundamental truth. Each cancer is different. Each diagnosis is different. There is no uniform way for coping, or treating, or dealing with this disease. Once I found that it was ok to cry the most amazing thing happened. I found that I could laugh again. Acceptance, just like I had learned the first time, was the key. Once I accepted that I once again had to fight, I found my laugh. (Small chuckles at first.) It seemed I had only forgotten for a little while. I had to learn some new lessons and I had to learn a few over again. I felt it important to share these lessons as if I had an obligation. If I can impart any advice, any wish for other survivors of whatever circumstance, no matter how bleak the future is I hope you never forget to take time to reflect and renew, and that you never forget how to laugh.

Foreword

I first met Lauren when she came to me in November 14, 2000. At that time she had been found to have a 2.5 cm. cancer of her left breast with metastasis to 8 of 14 axillary lymph nodes. She had already received 4 cycles of Adriamycin Cytoxan. From March through May of 2001, she was given a definitive dose of radiation therapy to her left breast and left supraclavicular fossa that she tolerated rather well.

Lauren did well for almost 2 years, but she was referred back to me in May of this year with a 2-week history of pain in her sternum and a CT scan showed extensive destruction involving her breastbone. Fortunately the PET scan showed only involvement in that area and in no other location. At that point Lauren was given additional radiation therapy over her sternum. The techniques used, i.e., electron beam caused a significantly painful skin reaction that took several weeks to clear. In time the radiation markedly reduced the pain, but not completely.

It's been my privilege to be involved with Lauren's care during the time that she required radiation therapy. Initially I saw her for breast cancer, and more recently metastasis to her sternum.

One of Lauren's many talents is the ability to write in descriptive detail her unplanned journey in dealing with this chronic disease known as cancer.

I found Lauren's first book entitled *"Don't Let The Cat Get Your Wig and Other Things the Oncologist Never Told You"*, to be highly informative and amusing. Her second book entitled *"That's So Funny I Forgot To Laugh"* (Facing a Cancer Recurrence) offers a unique insight into the personal experiences this young lady has had with not only the initial diagnosis of cancer, but what it is like to deal with recurrence, with the usual delay in the diagnosis, and the pain and anxiety that goes with having to deal with it. Anyone who has had anything similar to her experiences or their family will find this book to be informative and of some real comfort.

Timothy E. Cloninger, M. D.
President, Southeast Radiation Oncology

Chapter 1

It was Friday night. My husband pulled our loaded up Rav4 next to the curb at the bistro and I parked the new Accord in a proper space in the lot. The usual drill began as together we quickly started pulling musical equipment out of the back of our little SUV and setting it on the sidewalk before security came along to tell us we couldn't park there. People always marvel at the amount of stuff we can cram into such a small vehicle as if we are reminiscent of one of those little VW's that keep unloading clowns. I made a feeble apology for not being able to carry as much as usual due to this chest cold that was causing me quite a bit of pain. Scott, my husband and music partner, just nodded and said to go get the back door open so he could get everything in easily and without bothering the patrons. It was a regular gig for us, playing a jazz/eclectic mix for the dinner crowd and bar patrons who by this time knew our music very well. This was both our part-time job and passion. We considered most of them friends even though we hated to deal with the acoustics in the place.

I got the door and headed for the bar. Christian, my favorite bartender went straight for a bottle of Sauvignon Blanc before I interrupted his rhythm and asked instead for a coffee with some type of liqueur. I hoped it would smooth out my voice and the pain. He fixed me something hot with chocolate sprinkles on the top and smiled his wry sardonic smile. He said something sarcastic as usual, but since it's such a habit for him I forget exactly what. Everyone at the bar exchanged pleasantries and I told them I might not sing as much as usual tonight. I might rely on our guitarist for some instrumentals. No one seemed to mind as long as the music and the alcohol

1

kept coming. For most of the night I floated back and forth in front of the mike, singing as I felt like it, and clutching my chest in the corner when I didn't. Not really wanting to make a fuss. After all, I knew what *really* being sick was about and I didn't want to sound like a wimp. Besides anytime I do mention health issues to most people they just smile and remind me that they are just happy I am still here. Then I feel silly for complaining, not to mention a bit guilty.

Funny when we finished I got more compliments than usual on my voice. Maybe it was the liqueur, or maybe I just tried harder since I didn't feel as good. As much as I always enjoy the attention and compliments I was so tired that the effect was lost. I just wanted to go home, so I asked Scott if he minded. Of course he said no, even though I know it's difficult to load so much heavy equipment alone. I felt guilty…but not that guilty. He reminded me to be careful driving home. I wasn't sure it was me, or the new car he was worried about, but we were both treating it like a baby so I assured him I would use extra care. I hauled myself to the parking lot feeling the full brunt of the extra 20 pounds I'd put on in the last year and I drove straight home.

By the time I got there I noticed that damn chest pain again, more intense now, maybe because I was alone for the first time to sit and think about it. I didn't even go into the house. Instead I sat at the edge of the driveway, staring down the street, waiting for Scott to come home. My intention? To get him to take me to the emergency room as soon as he got there. At least I could get some antibiotics and painkillers. I had to do something; I'd ignored it long enough.

As much as I hate the emergency room, it was my only option at this late hour, and I didn't have time to make any more doctor visits anyway since I'd just started a new "day" job. I waited. Scott agreed. We both hoped it was a quiet Friday night with no drive by shootings and very few heart attacks to back up the wait. Selfish thoughts, but we were tired and I was in pain. Sometimes you can really get selfish when the pain gets bad.

The sliding doors opened and we were relieved to see a relatively small number of people. The receptionist behind the counter insisted on the gratuitous paperwork. It was obvious she didn't enjoy dealing with the public. It was also obvious that I hated that ridiculous paperwork. The same junk I've filled out by rote at this point more times than I can count. I took the pen and clipboard and we sat down as far away from anyone else as we could. Despite that fact in the next ten minutes a rather large boisterous family decided to sit right in front of us even though the room was almost empty. (I never understand that, it always happens at the movies too.) I moved my thoughts from my irritation to the form and filled out the name, social security number, and employment information. For a moment I thanked heaven above that my husband was not only an exceptional musician, but also a contractor for IBM. Our insurance, while not perfect, was substantial. I moved down the list of illnesses to check off. "Do you have a history of: Diabetes? No, High Blood Pressure? No, Heart Attack? No, Cancer?...Yes."

"Here we go", I thought, as I had to fill in the additional blanks requiring detailed explanations. "I always hate this part", I muttered to Scott, as if my whole previous breast cancer experience was an irritation like standing in line at the bank. It kept me from filling out the form fast enough to get in front of everyone else waiting to get medical attention. Besides, half the time I am frightened that doctors who don't know my history won't even bother looking at that section since I'm only 36. I might add I also don't look my age, another reason they would discount bothering to take me seriously. Grudgingly I finished the information and returned the form to the desk. Scott and I moved to the back corner of the room for some quiet and rested against each other. I apologized for dragging him out in the middle of the night for something so minor. He said he didn't have anything better to do and we stared at the silent TV.

When they finally called me back into a room they took my vital signs and asked the standard questions. They told me someone would be in with me shortly and they would want to do a Chest X-Ray and EKG. At least there was a plan, and I was so tired I started to lie back on the bed. Suddenly the pain was so severe that tears rushed to my eyes and I strained to get back upright. Scott saw the look in my eyes and did his best to assist me in sitting up. I was in extreme pain and it was a good thing I was there. Maybe I had developed some type of pleurisy. We didn't want to even think about pneumonia for a singer. That would truly mess up our already muddled finances and already booked gigs. We both began taking my symptoms a little more seriously.

I've never understood why they have to take a perfectly upright person in a wheelchair to X-Ray, but nonetheless I hopped on and allowed myself to be driven down the hall. I knew the X-Ray would show my recent ski-injury I sustained while flying over someone's abandoned poles on the slope at Snowshoe. It was the first time skiing so I had to break something. I told the technician, so they would be prepared. They snapped my little photos and sent me back to the room. The technician who did the subsequent EKG had to do it twice because somehow he got the charges reversed, or something like that. I sat up straight finally and watched the clock. It was around 1am when they came to tell me the tests were fine. I probably had severe inflammation. They gave me two Vicodin and some high dose Ibuprofen. By the time it kicked in I felt fine. They gave me a prescription for more to get me through the weekend. Thank goodness it was nothing serious. I wasn't happy about one more medical bill, but at least insurance would cover most of it and I could relax. I was told if the situation didn't improve to see my family doctor in about a week. "Fine", I muttered. I was sure I wouldn't need all that. Just some rest is all I needed. I was probably pushing too hard. No one even mentioned a pulmonary embolism, which I later found out was a complication of breast cancer survivors. I wondered if they even read my paperwork fully, but the Vicodin just made me want to curl up at home in my own bed, so that is where I went.

Chapter 2

I went back to my new job on Monday and sat in the sales meeting. There was a heated discussion going on involving commissions. I really didn't care. I was new, so it barely affected me, and I was on Vicodin, so *nothing* affected me. I coughed a bit and I don't think I looked very good. By the time the meeting was over the boss sent me home. It was obvious I wasn't myself. I fought it. I tried to work more during the week, but the heat from impending summer, the pain, and the drugs made me completely ineffective. At the end of the week my boss got fed up and called my family doctor. He convinced him to work me in as soon as possible, which unfortunately wasn't for a few days. I worked on and off trying to rest when I could. I feared I'd get so far behind I'd never catch up and I wanted so badly to have a fresh start and not screw this up. After the cancer I kept trying desperately to start over.

My family doctor or GP as they call them is a former client from a former advertising sales job. He is also an exceptional person, along with his nurse, Paula. It wasn't that anyone really had to force me to go see them, I just did not want to have to stop my schedule to make the long drive to find out nothing was really wrong. Nonetheless once I got there the visit was wonderful. I tried to catch them up on my life, my new job, and the music, everything that was going on. Everyone commented on how great I looked. Why in the world would anyone think I was sick? They kidded that I just wanted to visit. I was tan, a little bit heavier, but healthy looking. By all accounts they felt all I needed was perhaps an antibiotic to kick the stubborn bug and some more ibuprofen for the inflammation. Still as a precaution, as will always be the case for me, they wanted blood work. Just in case. Of course he did want me to stay home and rest for a day or so. I called the boss, who laughed at the big long word that meant inflammation (Costochondritis), and told him I'd work from home the next day.

The following morning as I sat with my day planner and phone in hand making appointments, my husband left a frantic message on our voicemail. He couldn't get through to me on the telephone because I was too busy making appointments for later in the week. It seems the doctor's office had to call him at work because they also could not get through at home and they needed to talk with me urgently. Apparently, there was something in my blood work that raised a concern. I was to call the office ASAP.

Once I mouthed off to myself about the inconvenience of being interrupted, I phoned the doctor's office. The assistant who answered tried to explain to me what the concern was but I could feel her exasperation. She was simply relaying a message. All she knew was that I needed a CT scan...today. What could possibly be the rush? Finally she asked if I wanted the doctor to call me. We felt that was the best solution for both of us so I waited in anticipation, shaken, but not severely. I called work and tried to tell them why I was going to the hospital for a test with the skeletal information I knew, then I took a hot bath to calm my nerves. In the midst of all of this my doctor called. "Lauren, its Ned", he said calmly. "They asked me to give you a call." He then told me of his fear for a pulmonary embolism (as mentioned earlier) and that my blood work was at a borderline level. He just wanted to be sure.

I relaxed. I didn't hear anything else except that it really wasn't as frantic as it sounded. It was just a precaution. I tuned out the other details then got dressed, called my husband away from work and headed to the hospital for the tests. We spent most of the drive over discussing where we would eat for dinner and how long we thought this would take.

It took a long time. One machine was down so they were backed up. It was an extensive wait in a waiting room with no reading materials, save a bookshelf with nothing but bibles. I'm a spiritual person but I found that a bit disconcerting. What were they saying? All you have is a prayer? Scott and I found ourselves discussing the lack of literature and the cute little old lady who was answering the same standard gratuitous questions I always hate. Only she was getting an oral exam by a medical assistant trying to admit her. I am sure the reason was that her eyesight made reading a challenge, but she cheerfully answered all the questions from the assistant as though she were as young and spry as a teenager. No major illnesses, but everyone in the room laughed when she was asked if she had any body piercings, such as her nose or belly button. Did they have to ask? It made the wait interesting until they finally called me back.

It was cold in the "holding" room where they left me with 3 other patients. The seats were hard and there was one window. Everyone shivered. I noticed there were drawers under the seats and opened one. I suspected there might be blankets or gowns in them. I was right. I wrapped 2 green hospital gowns around myself and tried to huddle myself against the wall. Scott was back in the original waiting room. I had no one for conversation. Fortunately they called me out of there first.

Unfortunately once they got me in the room for the scan they could not hit a vein. I distracted myself by marveling at how the scanning apparatus looked like a giant white doughnut. They injected me 4 times with no success before they put me back in the "holding" room and called the "IV" team. I chuckled to myself as I pictured men in black jackets with bold lettering on the back quickly racing to find a vein like some kind of NASCAR pit crew. I asked for Scott since I had to wait. They finally let us wait in another room where I could lie down. I waited and prayed I would not have to take much more needle torture.

Finally the "IV" team arrived or at least one member of the team. Not exactly as I pictured. It was a little lady named Scottie, who was very sweet and very direct with that needle. She succeeded on the first try and while it hurt like the dickens (due to the size of the needle), I thanked her profusely. She commented that she liked my shoes and I admit I was flattered, but all I could wish for on my feet at that time were insulated boots. I wondered why hospitals are so cold? We said our goodbyes; after all sticking someone with a needle is pretty personal. She left and another technician escorted me back to the scanning room.

They told me that the dye would cause a heat sensation throughout my body. To me the process was fascinating. I watched and waited to feel the warmth after being so cold for so long. I felt it. It was as if I drank hot liquid that spread not just to my stomach, but also through my entire bloodstream, and it felt wonderful. Well at least until it got to an unmentionable place. There the sensation of heat was a bit overwhelming and shocking. I teasingly told the technician he could have warned me. The only other time I had felt something like that is when I had used the shampoo instead of shaving lotion in a very sensitive area. All I wanted was cold water and I wanted it quickly (and I might add, not for drinking). My eyes bulged and I looked at my husband. I reminded him to ask me about that later, it was a little personal for discussion in front of the medical staff.

The machine even told me when to breathe and when not to, which is so different from something like a mammogram where the technician bears that responsibility. After I was done breathing on cue, they sent me back to the bible room where I waited once again. I wasn't sure why, I didn't think I would get the results that quickly. Then again the technician mentioned that pulmonary embolisms could be dangerous and sneak up quickly. I figured they wanted to be sure so we kept waiting. We had arrived at 3:30 it was now almost 7:00. Again Scott and I began discussing dinner when they called me back to the reception desk. I've spent a lot of time having medical tests in my life but this was odd protocol. The receptionist handed me the phone and my doctor was on the line. Once more I heard the familiar, "Lauren, its Ned", only it was followed by "Do you want to come by and talk?" In that instant I knew, it wasn't congestion, it wasn't inflammation and it wasn't a pulmonary embolism. The cancer was back.

In the parking lot on the way to the car I tried to prepare Scott for this news, but he wanted to hear from the doctor first. His protectiveness and his defense mechanisms would not accept it until he heard it directly. I don't want to sound sexist but I believe that is distinctly male. I believe my familiarity with my body and my female intuition are what told me before I was told, as it did with my initial diagnosis of breast cancer 2 years earlier. Something had told me then and something was telling me now.

Cliché as this may sound, the drive to the hospital seemed forever. The sun was setting and the world seemed strange and far away. The only thing I could think of other than how this was going to sound was that I was fortunate to have a physician who would meet me at his office at 7pm to discuss results of a test I just had that afternoon. Anyone who has dealt with cancer knows the agony of testing and waiting. If there was any bright side to this moment, this was certainly it. We pulled into the lot and knocked on the locked door. He met us fighting back tears.

I said, "Its back", he said "Yes". That's how I got the news. It had spread to my sternum. No wonder I was in pain, I had cancer in my bones. We all sat down on the sofas to get our bearings. It was hard for him, as he said he's not used to giving this kind of news. GP's usually refer questionable circumstances to oncologists who do tests. We both stumbled onto this diagnosis by accident but he said he had a gut feeling and had to follow it up. I thanked him and hugged him and I think that was bewildering. He had to tell a patient she had a cancer recurrence and the patient is grateful. What's even more bewildering is that in some way I felt more sorry for him. He had to go home after a long day and this was the last item on his agenda. What kind of sleep would he get, what kind of respite would his mind give him? I had family support because I was the patient. Who is going to support the doctor? He tried to call my oncologist who was unavailable at the time. Then we all grabbed some Kleenex and headed home.

The drive home was spent on the phone. I tearfully called family, friends and boss and tried to explain as much as I knew. It had spread but we didn't know how much. I didn't know treatment options yet and I didn't know when I would know. There were many other things I didn't know either. I didn't know that a recurrence automatically classified as a Stage IV cancer, the latest and most serious stage of development. I didn't know that I was now classified as incurable. One more thing I didn't know...according to most resources the 5-year survival rate was 20%. Not odds I wanted to see and not information you want to locate on the Internet at 2am alone in your bedroom. But that is precisely how and when I discovered how serious my circumstances were. This time things were different, less predictable and less favorable and I discovered that I couldn't escape the fear and pain no matter how hard I tried. During my previous treatment I had written a book advocating humor for healing, but I couldn't find my laugh. I remember looking at my husband and asking him "Where is my sense of humor?" His reply? "There's nothing funny about this."

That didn't stop me from searching for it. Forcing jokes and cracking puns, I tried to put that bravado back on. But the suit didn't fit anymore. I didn't want to be a hypocrite and I struggled mentally with that image of myself. I didn't even want to admit to writing the first book and I silently wished to myself I could take it off the market. Actually I was split down the middle on that. I wanted to continue to be proud of that accomplishment and believe that it had helped others; at the same time I couldn't seem to help myself. The book was a few years old and it stated in my bio that I was now in remission. Now that statement had become a lie. What could I do about that but go on about my business and fight the cancer once again. Images of chemotherapy, radiation and surgery danced in my head. I'd had all of those treatments to prevent this day from coming. It made me feel quite out of control. Of course I know control is an illusion, but I suppose its human to desire it. I admonished myself for asking to have my port removed, since I figured chemo was inevitable again. (The port was a device that delivered the drugs right to my bloodstream and made the needle pricks easier.) I looked at my arm, bruised and tender from the tests. I knew that seeing my oncologist would just make it worse. He would need even more blood work. The wait and see game had begun.

Chapter 3

Despite my disdain for ineffective and unobservant medical professionals, I have had the most wonderful and extensive care from my core group of physicians. I mentioned my GP earlier, but this group includes my oncologist and radiation oncologist. These caregivers have over the years almost become extensions of my family, so even given the circumstances I knew I was in good hands as I went for my exams and tests. When the morning of my first official recurrence visit arrived, I was at least happy to see the nurses and looked forward to, in a strange and anxious way, the attention from my oncologist.

Dr. Mitchell burst into the examination room where Scott and I sat, cold and frightened. He always makes a grand entrance. "Well shit!" he blurted, and I chuckled through my tears (The first clue that I would eventually be able to laugh again). He pulled out my chart and started reviewing information. He knew me well enough to know I'd ask a lot of questions so he went over the details he knew and we discussed early options and testing. Insisting that I get back on something that blocks estrogen and scheduling a PET scan and brain scan, he covered as much ground as possible as quickly as possible. The man is a speed demon and occasionally I have to slow him down to grasp everything. Not that I am slow, but it's always a learning process for me. So far the metastasis (spread, or mets for short) was only in the sternum, but we had to be sure. Consequently I got ready for the battery of tests. "Put your game face on", he said.

I had to wait almost 2 weeks for the tests. In the meantime
I had to decide what to do about the new job and I had to figure
out if I could handle the weekend gigs we had scheduled. I met
with my company and tried to work part time at first.   I
eventually agreed to take an unpaid medical leave due to the
stress, pain and eventual fatigue. Music on the other hand has
always been therapy for me. As long as my musicians knew I
might have to rely on them heavily to cover for me, I wanted
and needed to continue to sing. The play dates kept me going
and distracted but the pain was growing worse. I fought calling
the doctors for stronger painkillers, though I'm not sure why,
until finally I could not bear it anymore. By the time we
determined through the multitude of tests that the disease was
contained in the sternum, I was on Morphine. Vicodin didn't
touch the pain anymore and neither did Demerol.   They
prescribed 15 mg tablets and told me to take one every half
hour until the pain subsided. It was several hours before I
found relief. Then I had to struggle to keep the right amount in
my system. Eventually they prescribed 60 mg time-release
tablets in addition to the 15 mg to stop any breakthrough pain.
I was a walking zombie.

To my drugged out surprise chemotherapy was not
indicated for this treatment. A different form of radiation in a
3 to 4 week concentrated regimen was what was required. Dr.
Cloninger, my radiation oncologist explained how he would
use an electron beam to treat the area. I was a bit "out of it"
but I could tell as fond as we were of each other, he didn't want
to see me this way. His brow furrowed as he hugged me after
our initial consultation. At least it was our initial consultation
for the second time. He told me that I should experience some
pain relief almost immediately after starting treatment. That
was welcome news and I hoped it was true. I went home and

sent an email to my friends and family explaining what I knew. I'd been taking the morphine so I wanted to sleep, but knew I needed to eat. My mother made me some soup and I sat at the coffee table to force it down. Apparently I was quite humorous without knowing as I salted more of the table than my food. Who cared? I went to bed. For a good portion of my treatment, that's all I can remember. The radiation room for 5 minutes a day, and my bed for the rest.

A few weeks into treatment my Father-in-law invited us to Topsail Island. It sounded like a wonderful idea. A week away from all the mayhem in a relaxing environment could be such an escape. Only I was supposed to avoid the sun due to my increasingly angry burn, and I wasn't sure I could just take off in the middle of radiation therapy like that. I questioned Dr. Cloninger who assured me that I could use the rest and thought it sounded quite therapeutic. I spent the next few days planning and searching for a bathing suit that would cover up my treatment field, or as I affectionately called it, the "relief map of Italy" on my chest. I searched the Internet, but feared I wouldn't have time for anything to be shipped. Finally, in a little specialty swim shop, I found a "tankini" that zipped up the front all the way to my neck. It was adorable. It finally hit home that I was going on vacation…something I hadn't done in several years. The ocean was calling my name and all I wanted to do was sit on the beach and watch the waves pile into the shore. Wouldn't that be perfect?

Chapter 4

Well it was almost perfect. Scott's father was a great host. The weather held despite the occasional shower or storm. It should have been a great trip. So what was my problem? I was away from the "safety net" of my doctors and feeling nervous about leaving treatment behind. Even for a week. Perhaps it was an irrational fear, but whoever said dealing with cancer was rational. I was still on the morphine and though I had adapted, I still slept "in" on most days. Scott was on the other hand raring to go, and wanted his wife to be by his side. It created tension. He wanted companionship, and though I was right there with him, I felt incredibly alone.

There is nothing like the realization of your mortality to make you feel as though you are the only person on earth. No one can make that trip with you and no one can stop the inevitability that we will all leave this place someday. I looked for books of inspiration, but the stories fell flat as I sat on the beach and watched everyone going about with their lives. No one seemed to have a problem but me and no one would have looked at me and guessed. Nothing helped curb the fear of dying and the reality seemed so much more intense away from home and the familiar. What if treatment didn't work? What if there was more cancer somewhere else? How long do I really have? Pardon the expression, but these thoughts were killing me. Scott and I talked about it, then we fought, as fear breeds tension that has to be expressed. Then we talked some more. Then before I knew it, my trip was over.

I had wasted my opportunity to "get away". I had to return to reality. The truth of the matter however, was that I seemed to prefer reality. It was more comfortable to me. I was used to fighting, not sitting and thinking. I was ready to get home and back to treatment. It felt like I had an active role in coping and healing, rather than letting things happen to me. I felt safer in the hands of my physicians and my supportive family and I missed my menagerie of dogs and cats. Cats by the way, which had destroyed my curtains and completely redecorated the house by the time we got home. Martha Stewart has no threat from the feline community.

Back in treatment, I was told I could start weaning myself from the Morphine. I was almost done and the pain had significantly decreased. Easier said than done. As I tried I found myself somewhat chemically dependent on the drug. It was frightening to me but I began to understand the difference between being chemically dependent and emotionally dependent on something as strong as a narcotic. I could look at the bottle on my bedside table and not desire to touch it, but my body began doing contortions on its own until I complied. There were various uncomfortable side effects, mostly gastrointestinal, but the ones that kept me up at night were the "willies" as I called them. I kicked. I jerked and I twisted. Finally one night I gave in, positioned myself crosswise on the bed and began to kick as if I were in a pool for what seemed like an hour. The goal in my mind was to wear out my body until it could no longer go and I would force myself to rest from sheer exhaustion. It didn't work. I wound up taking morphine and sleeping the entire following day. I finally figured out that I could at least switch drugs and I could step down to Vicodin. I still had some pain so technically I needed something, and my body didn't seem to distinguish between narcotics. I shared this with my doctor who agreed that going totally "cold turkey" might not be in the cards for me just yet.

Chapter 5

I sat up from the radiation table for the last time…again. I took off the gown, dropped in the hamper, threw on my shirt and scurried out to the waiting room. I waived to the receptionist and motioned to my father, who went with me regularly, that I was ready to go. Even though radiation was always a fairly quick daily regimen, I surprised him with the speed in which I was able to get in and out on that last day. I was ready to be finished and move on, if that was indeed possible. In the car he asked if I wanted to go anywhere before heading home. "No", I said, "I just want to go to bed". There are two givens with radiation treatment. There's going to be"sunburn", and there's going to be fatigue. Between the drugs and treatment, sleep was better than chocolate. It was all I wanted all the time. I remembered being so tired from treatment 2 years prior and I had always thought the chemo had been the culprit. I began to realize that radiation had affected me more than I probably suspected.

I managed to do a few things in the weeks that followed. I wrote a bit here and there and busied myself around the house. I also began to plan for our 5th wedding anniversary that was to take place in October. I had wanted to wait until I was more confident with my treatment schedule before I started making plans. Having an event to look forward to became an obsession. It started out as a simple vow renewal ceremony and slowly began to turn itself into a fundraiser for breast cancer research. A friend from my hometown of Greensboro told me of a group she was working with, a grassroots effort to raise seed money for research. Instead of one more group searching for an elusive cure, this group designated funds to discover a test for breast cancer much like the PSA for prostate cancer. I knew that current diagnostic tools had limitations and I felt very strongly that the first step in curing a disease is knowing that it exists. I was overwhelmed with ideas and found that the project snowballed. It was big enough to get me excited but far enough away that I could still relax and plan slowly. At least at first.

A week passed, then two. The pain in my neck nagged at me. It seemed to be increasing. I mentioned it to the doctors on short subsequent visits and they assured me that it was leftover inflammation from the radiation. I accepted that explanation. I was almost too tired to care for a while. Still groggy from the treatment and the drugs, I continued to "sleep it off", as if the whole thing had been one big wild party and I had a month long hangover. I watched my hair grow too, as I had decided that if I didn't have to have chemo I wanted to see how long I could grow it again. Amidst all of this excitement it was time to start my new lines of therapy, Aromasin and Lupron. Basically the doctors referred to it as "chemical castration". The goal being to shut down my ovaries. You see fortunately for me my original tumor was "estrogen receptor positive" (er+). That means it fed on the estrogen my body produced. If you cut out the estrogen, you cut out the cancer's food supply. It is a positive sign if a tumor responds to estrogen as it gives you one more weapon with which to fight.

Unfortunately, I did not tolerate my first round with these drugs and after consultations with my doctors we decided against continuing the Tamoxifen. This time there was no choice. The cancer was more invasive than we had initially thought and we had to reinvestigate treatment options.

Scott and I had initially wanted children. I always pictured him as an excellent father. We clung to that possibility even after the first diagnosis. We knew then that there would be a risk. But over time we began to realize that I was aging, I had other health complications that might affect pregnancy and our lifestyles were not conducive to childrearing. Our music and work kept us from being home and we had come to realize that we enjoyed our lifestyle and the music too much to be able to stop. By the time they told me about this new treatment we had accepted that we might never have children of our own. Still there is a feeling of loss that we experienced, and as a female I knew that that was one part of womanhood I would never know. When you are faced with the permanence of that, it still leaves an impact on you. Watching as most of our peers became parents stung our hearts. We shared their joy but we ached for our own loss. It was however an unpleasant, but acceptable loss. You make your choices.

So I began taking the Aromasin for 2 weeks prior to the follow up visit where I would be given my Lupron shot. Basically the drugs work together to shut down my ovaries, much like a chemical hysterectomy. Of course there were side effects but they were generally mild. I began to notice night sweats, which created a laundry debacle. I had one good solid hot flash, much to Dr. Mitchell's delight. To him it meant the medication was working. To me it meant I needed a better fan in my bedroom. Actually I would get exceedingly hot and wear next to nothing. Then I would freeze to death and put on long johns. I can't say how many times I changed clothes in a day. It was like a little fashion show, only any makeup I managed to put on mostly sweated off my face. Oh yes and the acne was a nice addition. I had to take steps to correct that as well. I feared for the day when I grew a mustache. All of the signs of menopause were approaching and I hadn't even had the shot yet.

The Lupron shot didn't hurt, at least not when it first went into my left hip. But my neck was killing me. It had not improved. One afternoon while backing the car out of the driveway I managed to hit the garbage can because I didn't want to strain my neck to look too far behind. Yes Scott laughed at me, who wouldn't, but I knew it shouldn't be hurting like that. So on the day of the shot I whined to Dr. Mitchell that the pain had gotten more intense. Fortunately he's a doctor who listens so while I waited for my blood work to be done, he scheduled an MRI for later in the week. They put a band-aid on my arm and sent me on my way. My parents, who had once again come in for the doctor visit, joined us in the lobby and we headed off to lunch. We zipped over to a nearby grill that Scott had frequented for lunch during work hours. It was the first lunch I remember actually eating out and "desiring" since the craziness had started. Small things like that are so memorable and they symbolize a victory. Lunch like that before would have meant nothing, but this meant I was healing; moving on.

Scott had already taken so much time from work I thought I should go to the MRI alone. Then I thought better of it. I asked a friend to take me. Just the waiting can be unnerving. We watched a few minutes of Oprah as I filled out the paperwork that I love so much. I had been told to arrive at 3:50 for a 4:20 appointment. Just for the purpose of filling out said paperwork. I expounded on just how "efficient" I thought that process was when to my surprise they called me back early. Once again I dressed in the lovely green gown and made my way to the giant white donut that they call the MRI machine. "We are going to inject you with contrast" the technician informed me. I rolled my eyes. "I take it you don't enjoy that" he inquired. "Its just that no one can ever find my veins", I replied. He looked at me with doubt in his eyes and grabbed my arms. "Why you have great veins, that shouldn't be a problem. We'll get it on the first try" he quipped. I shrugged my shoulders and thought to myself "yeah right dude". Then I lay down on the table and stared up at the ceiling where someone had thoughtfully placed images of backlit trees and birds. I wondered if anyone really thought that would help when you are stuck inside a tube for 30 minutes listening what sounds like street construction all around you. "Here we go" he said and slid me back into the machine, handing me headphones as I went. I hope it's on a decent station I thought to myself.

For the first 30 minutes of the test no contrast was injected. I also quickly realized that the radio station didn't matter since I couldn't hear it over the clanging of the magnet. I thought back to my very first MRI when I had worn boots with metal zippers. I remember the machine trying to pull them inward and marveling at the strength of the magnetic force. I tried not to think about the upcoming needle experience until at last it was upon me. The technician asked me if I was on any medication. I chortled and then reeled off the list...Aromasin, Zoloft, Vicodin, Lupron, and Ativan. He tried to look at my left arm and I motioned him away. Clearly my response was not expected. I cannot have blood work done on that arm due to previous surgery and I even wear a medic-alert bracelet. They never notice. When he finally got to my right arm I tried to prepare him. "They roll", I said, referring once again to my ever-evasive veins. "Everyone's veins roll", he said. I braced myself for impact. I felt the needle go in and in. It rumbled around. I knew that feeling; he couldn't get it to feed the IV. "So far you called this right," he said. Unfortunately, I didn't want to be right, just done. "We use this area below your thumb as a last resort because it generally doesn't feel very good." Now there were two reasons I didn't want to hear that. I can surmise that it wouldn't feel good that close to a bone. I wasn't looking forward to it. Also someone had tried it before and failed. Pain with no result was not something I needed at this point. Mind you no one ever reads this on my face. I am always calm and quiet. I find it is the best way to cope. To my surprise he eventually did hit the vein. It took a moment, and the contrast burned. I wondered if I could stand another 30 minutes with that pain in my bone. Eventually it eased. Later than sooner the test was finally over and another technician informed me I could go. "Good", I said referring to the headphones, "I hate this song".

Chapter 6

That weekend was a long one. We had one gig at one of our favorite places, but we got rained out on the third set. Scott had also made plans to see his college buddies in Raleigh that weekend. I knew I wouldn't make it. Lately I had been nauseous in the car for any ride over fifteen minutes. I also knew that after playing I'd have no energy so I knew I'd have to disappoint him and ask to remain home for the trip. Since I knew this would upset him I stewed about it for hours until marching downstairs and announcing rather angrily that he shouldn't expect so much from me. My approach was a little over the top and was met rather gruffly. It was a long night. Finally he told me he suspected I probably couldn't handle it. All I wanted to know was why didn't he just come and say that to me. Instead of letting me think I somehow had to force myself. Then I realized that this could be a male/female thing and we finally went to bed. He took off for Raleigh early in the day. I stewed in my juices until he called that night and we finally worked it all out for good.

It was a good weekend for Turner Classic Movies. I watched Gone With the Wind, Love Affair, Affair to Remember and Dark Victory. Dark Victory...I remembered seeing the ending of that movie years ago. I knew it probably wasn't a good idea to watch it. Bette Davis dying of a rare cancer at a young age is not exactly escapism for a cancer patient. But I did. I watched the whole thing. And at 6am exhausted, bleary eyed and scared witless, I went to the bathroom and looked at my neck, where I believed I saw swelling. Was it real? No it couldn't be. 10 minutes later I went back and stared again. No...there's nothing there. Is it?

This agony went on for hours until I finally called my parents in Greensboro. They were scared witless too; I really shouldn't have frightened them. It's just that I could see something, I thought, but I wasn't sure. It was obvious to them I hadn't rested. They knew I had morphine left and suggested I take some. I looked at the bottle and it looked at me. Then I took some and about lunchtime I felt weird and sleepy. So I went to bed. I slept until Scott came home and awoke with the worst headache I could imagine. He offered to make me some soup so I could take a pain pill. I wandered downstairs. He said he thought he could see something on my neck too. Maybe I wasn't crazy.

Once downstairs I realized food wouldn't make it to its final destination. I threw up the soda Scott had given me. I tried to eat the soup and threw up all 3 spoonfuls. Then I began throwing up nothing. I tried a Phenergan, always good for first level nausea. I threw it up. I tried another and threw it up. After throwing up the 3rd we called the doctor who called in some Ativan. I had taken it before and it always helped because I could place it under the tongue. Once I got the Ativan, the discomfort eased. Lying on the bathroom floor sweating was almost like going through chemo again. I stared at the familiar crevices in the floor and I decided that no matter how much pain/fear I am in, morphine just isn't something I want to take without supervision again. The after effects are far too extreme. Being that ill is frightening and horrible. At least I didn't think too much about those MRI results, not until the next morning.

The appointment was early enough, but the office was busy so we had to wait. We stared blankly at each other. We looked to see if we could still see any swelling on the side of my neck.

We decided we couldn't. One of the nurses said the doctor was on his way. We exchanged a look of dismay interpreting that as a statement of delay. Dr. Mitchell of course finally bounded through the door as usual and instead of telling us any results simply hands me the paperwork. "I knew she wouldn't believe me unless she saw it for herself" he beamed. There was no evidence that the cancer had spread. I felt relieved and happy…and stupid. But the pain was still there and it was pretty extreme, what could it be? He suggested it might be arthritis possibly due to the hormonal treatments or some inflammation from the radiation treatment and nerve damage. "Its not in your head" he said. Well I knew that. I knew it wasn't psychosomatic but I didn't really have a reason to hurt like that. I felt bad for needing the pain pills. Well not bad enough to give them up. Every time I tried the resulting pain was almost debilitating. Cancer would have explained it. Now I feared I'd cried wolf for no reason. I only hoped that next time I did so, I would still be taken seriously.

I left feeling relieved and disturbed, just like I did when I first found that lump several years ago they said was probably fibrocystic. They were wrong then. Should I still be worried? Should I take the results at face value? If I have an 80 percent chance of recurrence in the next 5 years, what is it going to feel like and how do I find it. How seriously do I take every ache and pain in my body. I'm supposed to be relieved now, I'm supposed to be laughing again…all I had were more questions. I would just have to wait and I would have to learn to laugh while I did so. I decided could live with that and right now it looked like I was going to live, for a while anyway and that was more of that time I had begged God for. Scott and I ate lunch, and started making some plans.

Chapter 7

The doctors really didn't want me back in the workaday world just yet. I wasn't totally out of the woods. We could just see the clearing. They also really didn't want me back in the field I had been in due to the stress level. Everyone knew music was my first love and therapy, so Scott and I decided to try to put together a different musical project. One that would get us more work and possibly pay some bills in the meantime. I wondered about disability. I was told I couldn't get it my on my first experience with treatment. Still I recovered well enough with only few lingering side effects. The fatigue being the most prominent. I started doing research into getting assistance and found confusion staring me in the face. If I looked at my prognosis on paper or the Internet, all the resources for me were "end of life" issues, dealing with wills and acceptance. That isn't where I felt I was, even though the facts and figures supported it. According to my doctors though, they felt sure that they could isolate this particular recurrence and eradicate it totally. Then with the hormonal treatments prevent future recurrence. Who do I believe? What a frustrating mumbo jumbo. I realized that there wasn't any material that really addressed someone like me. Someone perhaps who is stage 4 but with a better prognosis. I started writing again not only to tell my story but also provide other material to women (and men) with metastasis besides directions for filling out their will and testament. I knew I needed to attend to that, but I was busy living at the moment and I intended to keep it that way. If I could share music and hope, I'd be doing my life's work. I set about doing just that.

That theory was excellent, but the reality was that days ran together.   During this period my sleep schedule became irregular. My moods did too. An important gig got cancelled due to severe storms; the second in a week. I needed the money and I needed the diversion. I tried to write, mostly in the dark at 3am. Some of it was therapeutic, some of it was just rambling. I tried to keep myself from slipping into depression, but it was difficult. I kept feeling that pain in my neck. Sometimes more intense than others. It never let me forget for long how different my life was than that of my peers. I could accept it, but it was hard to interact. No one really knew what to say, and most conversations with others my age sounded like tripe. I guess I was a cancer snob. I just didn't think they could get it, but sometimes I felt it was my job to try. Many times I drew new people into my life. Sometimes I alienated them, but I was doing my best to make a difference in the world for as long as I could.

Many thoughts crossed my mind in the waiting period before the final tests could be performed. I could have been a better daughter, wife, pet parent or citizen.   I could have studied something else in college or gone back to school. What if I could start fresh? What would I do? What things could I take care of that I had left undone? Sometimes those thoughts were so overwhelming that I found I actually did nothing. I lay in bed and didn't answer the phone.   It was usually bill collectors anyway, what could I tell them? I had no answers. All I knew is that I had to do something, anything each day to ease forward and somehow I managed to do so.

The Pilates program I ordered off the Internet helped me stay focused, though I felt it was a little too easy to really give me the results I wanted. I chose it because it was low impact.

I also knew I had to do something to take advantage of the steroid I had been put on to fend off the cancer. Dr. Mitchell was most excited to see if I could "buff up". Each visit to the office required me to show off a bicep. If there was a positive to all this, I looked like I was in fantastic shape. Between my abs and the self-tanner, no one would guess my inner turmoil and I took almost a sick pleasure in that. I might have been struggling but dammit honey I looked great. I darkened my hair to cover the gray that snuck up on me. My husband chased me all over the house and that I truly loved. (Even if I had no sex drive at all…which of course was to be expected.) The hot flashes increases and I prayed I wouldn't grow a mustache. I found to my dismay one evening a long black hair that I had to shave off my chin. I told no one.

Chapter 8

I started bulking up a bit and was enjoying incredible abs without as much work as usual. It got addictive. The more I worked out the more I wanted to workout. Unfortunately I was getting headaches on top of the already aching neck. I attributed them to the Zoloft I was on, so I backed off of the drug a bit. I absolutely hated being on so much medication. We'd been rained out of so many gigs that when I finally got to play one Saturday afternoon, I found myself worked up. I was more than worked up really. I was angry that there wasn't much help for women my age with cancer, angry that there was little understanding, and angry about a certain venue that wasn't booking us anymore. I left the house in that state. Instead of pulling up looking "suave" in the new car, I accidentally bumped someone who had parked sideways in the spot I was attempting to park in. No damage to their vehicle but a clip in my front bumper. I told Scott. He was furious. I hid downstairs in the club with a glass of wine. When I tried to return to actually do my job and perform we were already testy with one another.

I decided to try to put out some flyers for the fundraiser and maybe rectify a misunderstanding with a nearby club. It was a way for me to feel productive and avoid Scott for just a while until things calmed down. That sounded like a good idea in theory but it didn't really work. I came back more frustrated than before due to the odd management of the aforementioned club. I glared at Scott. I tried to sing. The anger burned through my veins. I couldn't hear myself. A common complaint and one that I knew I had to ride hard. It was so common patrons used to come tell me. Only this time we had gotten new equipment and I was unused to the set up. Apparently people really could hear me. I was just used to the fight. When I turned around to discuss it with Scott again he hissed at me. The last straw. I picked up my purse and made a beeline for the car. Right in the middle of the set. Something I don't believe in, but I couldn't help my self. Seething, I peeled out of the parking lot and drove halfway of the short distance home. I then realized how unprofessional I was being. WHAT had come over me? I turned around. As I rounded one curve almost back to the venue I hit the curb, lost control of the car and totaled the brand new Accord against a tree. I sat motionless. Not only could I not make things better for myself, I had made them worse.

The ambulance came and I tried to explain whey they couldn't take my blood pressure from my left arm. Despite that medic alert bracelet I wear. They wrapped my painful neck, weak from cancer treatment in a protective device that nearly sent me to the moon. I tried to explain. "Cancer, I have cancer, it's in my chest and neck." It took many tries to get that across. The police had to go stop the band. Miraculously we were almost finished and the club understood. Well as much as anyone could. The club owner told my husband, "Its all those drugs she's on". They were most likely right. I remember an ex boyfriend of mine who used to be a body builder. He told me how when he used illegal steroids he used to have a hair trigger. He was constantly in a fight. I was on steroids now and I'd just shaved a hair off my chin. Why wouldn't they affect me the same way? And I hadn't taken the antidote because it gave me a headache.

Once in the hospital, I ripped off the neck device and looked around. Scott came in and I started sparring with him.

The nurse asked him to leave. A friend of mine sent her mom in with me and she was a godsend. She watched over me like a hawk. I was sent for more x-rays. I pleaded with the nurses to "find something". I kept thinking maybe they would find more cancer and it would explain that ongoing pain in my neck. They probably thought I was nuts. I wanted justification for my complaints. After being wheeled back in from x-ray I was given some Ativan and told I could get dressed. The doctor wanted to be sure it wasn't a suicide attempt. That was so far off base I laughed in his face. Only someone who wants to live is that angry at the possibility of death.

Once that hurdle was overcome we were almost clear to leave. I had allowed Scott back into the room along with my friend's mom. A knock on the door jolted me as I was dressing. I asked for a moment to prepare and motioned for the visitor to come in. Instead of the police officer who originally told me and my husband I was not charged with anything, it was a young boisterous cop who seemingly had an issue with me. He stormed in ranting about the tree that I destroyed and the skid marks on the road and the eyewitness he had. I was shocked. I tried to explain that I was in cancer treatment and the drugs…"**Cancer had nothing to do with it**," he said, "My uncle died of cancer". I may have been shocked but I certainly wasn't going to be talked to in such a manner. "Sir", I said to an officer likely 10 years my junior, "with all due respect cancer has everything to do with it." I tried to be respectful but he wanted a confrontation. So we let it be what it was. I was charged with reckless driving. When I was finally dismissed for home, my friend's mom offered to write a letter to the police chief. No, I said, I prefer to do it. Once again I felt it my job to speak for others. Sometimes when we make mistakes cancer is the driving force behind it. Others might not

Lauren Brower

be so vocal and no one deserves that type of treatment. My letter follows:

August 3, 2003

Dear Police Chief _____,

Dear Sir,
It is with great regret that I feel I must proceed in this manner, but I am writing to inform you of the offensive manner of one of your officers, _____. Perhaps he is an excellent officer and takes his job seriously. He did not lay a hand on me and in no way was physically abusive, but his words will stay with me forever and I find that I MUST write to inform you the effect that a statement such as his can make.

I was involved in a car accident on August 2nd. Whatever the results of that case may be the fact remains is that also I am a cancer patient and survivor. I say this not for your pity. I do not expect it or want it. I am now a stage 1V patient with metastasis to my bones. I am only 36 years old. I have a 10 to 20% chance of living 5 years. Perhaps the officer was unaware of the disease progression. Many are not when they view me by age. But I am unfortunately very sick and on medications that may affect my judgment.

When the officer almost forced himself into my hospital room (I was changing), he barely introduced himself and began telling me what happened in the events of that evening. Some of the story he tried to tell

38

was not entirely accurate. My first instinct was to try to explain my situation to him and that we may have to work to get the truth out, since I was indeed on several medications. I at that time said, "I have cancer so..." and was promptly cut off. Officer XXXXX informed me **"Cancer had nothing to do with it."** *He then informed that he just lost a relative to cancer. (I've lost many family members myself; it isn't the same as having it.) His tone towards me matched that of someone being questioned for child molestation. With all due respect, I wrecked my own car and hit a tree.*

Sir, there may be many things that I do not know. I know that college didn't prepare me for any of this, but I can tell you in all honesty that cancer has EVERYTHING to do with just about EVERYTHING I do every day. And I don't dwell, and I stay positive. (I even wrote a book). So If I may disagree with your officer, cancer affects me from the moment I wake up to take a pain pill, to what I wear and if I can get it on comfortably, to if I will be able to get out and run errands that day, or if the fatigue will keep me in bed. It affects the songs I listen to, the movies I see, the way I treat my loved ones and how long it will take me to fall asleep at night. Sometimes I get angry and confused. I look perfectly healthy, but I assure you the cancer affects more than you know. And while I am truly sorry for the loss of the officer's family member, I doubt he can make that determination without actually hearing me out. That he was that cold and crass to me is done. I hope he doesn't use that tone again to another survivor who might be less vocal but every bit as hurt. To a sick person, that is an abusive tone.

I know of no other way to explain to you how insensitive a remark like that is, but to say I did lose sleep and try to figure out how someone could be that cold. IF I made a mistake, which hasn't really been determined, I am sure that will be rectified. I will hear his words forever. I don't think that can be repaired. Not for me.

Sincerely,

Lauren Brower

I also sent a copy of the flyer for my fundraiser upcoming in October. I thought perhaps it would give them an idea of what the many faces of cancer might be. I also secretly dreamed that the police chief would make that rather pompous officer work security for the event. I knew that dream wasn't about to come true. I'll be lucky if I ever get an apology. But I shared my viewpoint and that's all I can do.

Chapter 9

I didn't want to see the car and I ached for what I had done. I let Scott handle the details and my family. We were lucky enough to get a rental of a sexy Chevy cavalier. It was awful. But it was a car and I was truly impressed with my insurance company. I didn't go anywhere for days anyway. I was embarrassed, sore and I didn't feel like doing anything. Our music was dying. I had just helped kill it. I had no other income and couldn't go get a job for not knowing what my health ultimately would be. Each day I felt a new pain. I tried not to be depressed but it was overwhelming. Scott nudged me back on the Zoloft. I finally painted my face 2 days later and we went to dinner. It was a start.

I was doing somewhat better until I decided to crochet a baby blanket for a friend who was due any second. I thought it would relax me. I couldn't put it down. By the time I finished it was almost daylight and I had cried over the thought of the new young life that would soon lie in it cuddled up new to the world. I ached that I would never have a child and that I myself was not that "new". That I might not have that much time left. I wanted to be that child, nestled warm and cozy and secure. Although I know security is an illusion, I cried till dawn.

Scott noted my complaints of pain continued. I think he grew weary of them. I didn't mean to complain, but leaning over to answer the phone in the morning caused just enough discomfort to deter me from doing it. Same with loading the dishwasher. It wasn't excruciating, I just wasn't getting anything done. I was fine if I just sat still. What kind of life is that? I also wasn't sleeping. I had the occasional nightmare about the accident. Not that I would die, but that I would ruin my reputation as a reasonable woman, a spokesperson and advocate. I didn't want to be the crazy mad woman who lacked self-control and ran around like a Looney. I decided the Zoloft was worth the headaches and hoped I hadn't done irreversible damage. Scott called the doctor and forced some tests to be scheduled. I was secretly relieved but didn't want to be difficult. They also prescribed some Ambien. One more drug to add to the collection. But I wasn't sleeping, maybe it would help. I kept having hot flashes…or power surges as my lady friends call them. Scott almost experienced one with me one night while seated beside me. He felt the heat radiate off me and thought he'd had one by default. At least it was some male sympathy. The laundry continued to pile up.

My parents had come into town to worry about me in closer proximity. I was glad they were here. But I was embarrassed too. Their daughter should have more self-control. Then I came to a new realization. If all this is hormonally driven as they say, telling me to "just control" my anger is like telling me to "just not menstruate". It's a little more complicated than it seems and I needed to allow myself room to cope. So in between fits of self-loathing I soothed myself with that. And I worked on writing, and getting my first book on tape. Anything I could do to redeem myself and help others. My goal and therapy was to focus on others. I knitted another baby blanket for a nurse at one of the doctor's offices and I started to learn a little Italian to surprise the folks at my favorite restaurant. I watched the skies to see if we were going to get rained out again and we kept trying to put a band together that would play indoors from now on.

I came to the conclusion that I would have to file for disability, whether I got it or not. I feared that process for many reasons. The stigma, my lack of steady work history due to illness and hearing that some examiners are known to be challenging. My phone appointment was coming up, and I was very, very nervous. I chose the phone appt. because I feared if they saw me they wouldn't believe I was sick. I looked fine. The external was an illusion I would have to overcome. But I couldn't find half of what they said they needed. Evidence of disease??? Should I show them by bones? What do they want? I could only stress about it for brief periods at a time. Then I would have to stress about something else. I'd go back to knitting again. This time a blanket for the chemo room. It was always cold in there.

Meanwhile Scott had made these appointments for me and I was going to have to explain the accident to Dr. Mitchell. Every little ache and pain intensified. Do I mention them to the doctor or no? Do I ask for help with the disability forms or no? Does he really know all the drugs I'm on? Well I couldn't just sit and dwell I had some time on my hands. The kind of time I hated having. Limbo. I dug out the Italian lessons and started working. Io Voglio...the first phrase I learned. "I want"...

How appropriate.

Chapter 10

There were a lot of sleepless nights waiting for those upcoming tests. Ambien helped a little. I could sleep in spurts. I was also nervously anticipating that call from the disability office. How would I be perceived? I struggled to accept that place in the world and to find a new identity. I didn't like driving past the scene of the accident. I hated myself for the person these drugs seemed to free from within me. Dr. Mitchell recommended I begin to see someone and I waited for his follow up call. I guess they were busy. I realized I'll have to do a lot of that work myself and I would have to instigate that procedure. No one could hold my hand to help me recreate and uplift my identity. I would have to do it myself. Time to rebuild from the ground up, not just redecorate.

If I could fill 15 pages of blank emptiness here to illustrate how the time dragged between doctor visits and tests and the answers that we always want I would. But you would just flip past them and it would be a waste of paper. But there were many days of imitating my housecats. Sleeping and running to the door for whatever purpose we didn't know. Playing for distraction and sleeping again. The silence can be maddening as it only allows you to think your thoughts. I envied the cats, they thought only of the pretty pink ribbon they chased all over the house. I thought it ironic that their choice of toy was indeed a pink ribbon from one of my shirts. Daily they would bring it into the room and lay it on the bed and look at me. They carried it everywhere. There was no escape. A strange metaphor.

The social worker from the oncologist's office called and set an appt. with me. At first I was half asleep when she called due to my messed up schedule, but when she called back later in the afternoon, I was thankful. It was a relief to talk to someone who understood the emotional impact of some of this, not just the medical approach. I am a member of an online support group and while extremely helpful it isn't the same. She made an appointment for the following week. I found myself looking forward to it. I felt that Scott was growing weary and not really understanding where all these emotions were coming from and God knows I'd dumped on my peers who just because of their life experience "couldn't get it". It almost sounds selfish, but I looked forward to going and talking about MY TREATMENT and ME without having to make apologies for it. Truthfully I couldn't wait. Even if I had to drive across town, which I had begun to hate. She could also help me file for disability, a big plus. My first interview had gone well enough, but most people need assistance with that process.

On top of all of this Scott had jumped up one Sunday morning and announced that he wanted to turn our bonus room into an "official" home studio. Normally a redecorating challenge is something I live for, unfortunately due to my waning energy I was less than enthusiastic. I let him start without me. But then my mind started running all the possibilities in my mind and the next thing I knew was painting an accent wall and retiling the floor. When I get started on a project like that I can't stop, so there were nights I went to bed at 2 and 3am and couldn't even function the next morning. Maybe I shouldn't have been doing it, but it did distract me. More than anything else had. Of course in the back of my mind, I wondered if I'd be around to really be able to use it.

How much music would I really be able to make there. Those thoughts just wouldn't go away. Damn them. I never mentioned them to Scott. I just kept painting.

Chapter 11

The night before the test results were to be given, we had a little snafu with our upcoming weekend band gig. After handling that crisis we had dinner. Then I went to bed. Chilled, I hovered under the bedspread and two blankets. I drifted,
slowly.

Tick...
Tick...

The clock said 12:39. I squinted at it across the room just to be sure. I had a hot flash and kicked all the covers to the floor, threw my arms across the bed and waited for the cool air to cover me. In 30 seconds I was shivering, I dug for the blankets from the floor with my sore neck and tried to drift again.

Tick...
Tick...

I lay at the foot of the bed with my face in the fan. My legs uncontrollably flailed or kicked again like I was in some strange body of water. I was half awake half asleep, but one thing I was not doing was sleeping.

Tick...
Tick...
Gave up on the foreign end of the bed and checked email. Funny no one was writing much at 3:45am. Lots of opportunities to meet local singles though, and several *can't miss* business opportunities that found themselves at the mercy

of my delete key. *"Hot hungry teenage girls looking for me?"* I don't want to feed these children. Let them go to the Waffle house, they can get a cheap meal there and it's always freezing. That should cool them right off. Meanwhile, I wasn't sleeping. Cancer patients and the Internet never sleep. Unless as you know, there's Morphine involved.

Tick...
Tick...

Mom? Are we there yet? I pulled out a book from my childhood. "Dr. Suess' Sleep Book". What a pleasant memory and distraction. Until I had a hot flash and had to kick off the covers. But by the end of the book I was cold again and felt tucked in. I took an Ativan and drifted off for a few minutes...

9 am found me exhausted. There were circles under my eyes that couldn't be covered by concealer. I ladled down the coffee my parents had brewed. I wouldn't have had the energy to make any on my own if they hadn't. I dressed warmly for the doctor's office and carried a little personal fan my mother had given me for the increasing hot flashes in my purse. The drive was surprisingly short and my father immediately hit the candy dish in the reception area in his usual childlike fashion.

I was called back to the examining area rather quickly but Dr. Mitchell was delayed. The nurses kept coming in to tell me he would be in shortly, which I knew to mean something was keeping him even longer. I knew the delays were unavoidable, but it made the wait almost unbearable.

My parents were with me, but Scott was at work and was listening in by cell phone. When the good doctor walked in he found me sitting on the table with a cell phone in one hand, a hand held fan in the other covered in the crocheted blanket that I had brought from home. It had to be a priceless picture and the laughter softened the mood. Then he said a word that I didn't expect to hear, certainly not in the context that he gave it.

NED…No Evidence of Disease. My scans, he said, were "beautiful", if a scan can be. I blinked in disbelief. Ned to me was a guy I used to know that smoked "a little something" on the side. "Ned the head" we called him. I didn't think it was a medical term but it was a fabulous word to me that day. Immediate relief swept over the room, but the questions still lingered. What is this pain? Why is it increasing?

I was told that I had necrosis in the area that was treated with the radiation. When my father asked about the palpable lumps that were still visible on my sternum again it was part of the same condition. I didn't ask much about necrosis because I was so relieved the word wasn't cancer. I still had the pain, but I still had time.

Dr. Mitchell referred me to a clinic to assist with the pain and wanted to change my antidepressant from Zoloft to Effexor because it might help with my other symptoms. I was ready to get rid of the hot flashes and sleepless nights so I was amiable to the change. I was so dulled from hearing the good news I left his office stunned. "What just happened? Am I ok? I'm ok! Now what?"

Chapter 12

I'd asked that question before after my first treatment and remission. "Now what?" It's almost as though there is a pressure for life to return to its pre-cancer state. But that is a complete impossibility to anyone who has had the disease. Metaphorically, Hurricane BC had whipped through my life a second time leaving in its wake emotional instability, financial insecurity, physical pain and an uncertain future. All that before I'd truly had the chance to rebuild from the first storm. Along with the relief came a flood of other emotions; shock, fear, anger, grief. Things that hadn't surfaced because I didn't have the time to focus on them. I'd been too busy fighting to analyze how I would feel when I won the battle. What battle had I truly won? If I keep fighting the battles will I ever actually win the war?

A war that seemed to mirror the current political situation our country faced. Attacked viciously and fighting an ever morphing invisible enemy that will probably never truly go away. It must be fought in different locations with different tactics until the end. There is no real victory for either side, there is just the battle and the end.

That may seem to sound a bit melancholy and even sad but the realization makes it easier to see that trite as it may sound we must learn to enjoy the journey, I must learn to enjoy my travels and not seek the end of the road. Learning to be present is a constant process and I believe the cancer returning taught me new lessons and new ways of coping. It taught me that I am not invincible, that I need to be reminded to cherish life yes, but not to be reckless with my attempts to embrace it.

I was invited sing in the mountains of NC on the weekend after I had been given the news. Instead of being so focused on the job and getting to the event to work, I actually enjoyed the drive. The weather was perfect, with the hint of fall approaching. When we arrived I said to Scott with slight abandon, "Lets stay the whole weekend, we have no other plans". And just like that our host offered to extend our stay, the rental car company let us keep the car until we were ready to return it, and the weather promised to be beautiful for the duration. As if the planets were all aligned, I felt there was a purpose in that trip. I felt that I was where I should be and that I was learning to enjoy where I was and not dwell on the future or the past. A difficult but rewarding balancing act.

I could continue to write about my experience with pain management as it moves forward. I could give detailed information about Necrosis and Costochondritis as I learn what it entails. I could even hash out every side effect of every medication that I am prescribed along the way, but I think I'll leave the story here, where it is open. That is the message that is coming through loud and clear. The story is never over. I'll leave the future for pondering, but the present for its lessons. The musings that follow are for that purpose; pondering and reflection, but not for dwelling and lingering.

In no way do I mean to insinuate that this experience is over. I continue to learn more about the after effects of cancer treatment every day. My husband and I have begun to show signs of marital distress, though we believe we can work through it and make our marriage stronger. Friends continue to come into and out of my life, which I understand is quite common. People will surprise you with their ability to understand, and some will surprise you when they just can't quite get it. So though I leave the story here, its far from over.

Dare I say I continue to learn to find the laughter through the pain. I crashed the class reunion of the graduating class before me because I realize you just never know how much time you have. Let us all dance while the sun shines. I wish for all those who have followed me on this diversion the same. Just don't forget to laugh along the way.

Epilogue

Some time after concluding the last chapter I waited on approaching a publisher to make sure that I had not overlooked information of relevance. One evening as I was surfing the Internet I sent Scott out for a chicken sandwich. I was on new medication and it was all I felt like eating. It was a craving I'd had for several days. My husband likes spicy foods and I needed something "normal" for a change.

Scott called me from his cell phone on the way home with surprising news. While standing in line for my sandwich he had encountered the original police officer from the evening of my accident. The one who said I would not be charged with any violations. They recognized each other, as they began to talk the officer began to apologize for his young colleague's behavior. The older officer apparently even told his "badge heavy" counterpart that he was wrong to have approached me in that manner. He also said he felt strongly that the case would be dropped. Apparently I am not the first person to have been treated harshly. When Scott called me to tell me this, I cried out of sheer relief. I only wished I had been there to thank him. The young officer's words would stop haunting me now. Even though at press time the case is still pending and may go to trial, I sent out for a chicken sandwich and got a side order of peace of mind as well.

Shortly thereafter, I celebrated my 37th birthday by doing what I love most, singing of course. Everyone thought I was crazy to ask to work on my birthday. My family was by my side as well as an amazing show of friends and supporters that also almost moved me to tears. Believe it or not, this time the audience actually sang happy birthday to the singer. My 35th birthday was the first after my previous treatment and I had looked forward to celebrating it. Unfortunately that date was September 12, 2001. My joy was dampened. My 37th birthday was the best celebration I can remember. Not only because I had such support around me, but also because I had the possibility of 37 more birthdays to look forward to.

Here's to the future. Here's to a cure, and a day when cancer no longer is a reason for young women to write books. Here's to laughter and to health for all.

Poems

I AM NOT FINE

*Just because I tell you
the words you want to hear,
it does not mean my mind
is completely free of fear.*

*Just because I put on
the face you want to see,
it does not mean reality
isn't frightening to me.*

*Just because I handle
my daily tasks at hand,
it does not mean I'm ready,
that I won't falter as I stand.*

*Could it be that you
are afraid that I'm not fine,
and I force you to face
the fears in your own mind...*

LB

TO SAY

Living at high speed,
Typing indeterminable words in the dark,
Waiting for wisdom, sweating in the interim.
Praying for brilliance to find me.

I feel the beast closing in, gnawing on the bones.
The urgency chokes me,
I think of nothing worthwhile to say.

Still I know that words may be my legacy,
All that will remain of what I am and know
...and don't know.

Quickly I must say something important,
pertinent, uplifting, inspirational and wise.
No pressure.

What have I learned?
That life isn't fair, womanhood is pain and joy,
Sleeping in is heaven and laughter is golden.
That cancer kills...

I cannot let it close in yet,
I still have not been brilliant.
I still have something to say.
I cannot die until I spit it out,
Until I fulfill my purpose.

I still have something to say damn it,
I still have something to say...

LB

MORNING FEAR

Through strange dreams
The sunlight beams
Across my weary eyes,
And morning turns
The lights on
Across the darkened skies.

And the trees whisper
They call my name
My purpose hidden
In their wicked game.

Tasks for all creatures
Come with the dawn
But for my life
Understanding is gone...

And the neighborhoods laugh
And the telephones tease,
The answers I search for
Still whispered by trees...

What do I do?
Why am I here?
I cry and cry back
Through my morning fear.

The sunlight poetic
Sparkles on grass
I would turn it off,
Let this moment pass...

No choices to make...
No future to fear...
I'd be back in my mind,
So strange and unclear.

But I lack such power,
And the trees...
They still talk,
So through the misty future
I stumble,
I walk.

LB

IN THE TWILIGHT

In the twilight
Of lost dreams
I lay awake and hear the restless souls.
I join in their chorus,
Our pain sings night songs.
Crying and wishing,
Crying and wishing.

In the streams
The sorrows flow,
The gurgling bubbling gushing of loss,
Of innocence and dreams,
Of a future now a past,
Dreaming and dying,
Dreaming and dying.

Wanting for better
But living with worse
I would not change my time here,
But hope that I
Have learned my lessons
Living and learning,
Living and learning.

Crossing the bridges,
Walking the paths,
Of new journeys of the heart and head,
I miss youth
But would not have it,
Burning and yearning,
Burning and yearning...

63

Lauren Brower

Crying and wishing,
Dreaming and dying,
Living and learning,
Burning and yearning...

LB

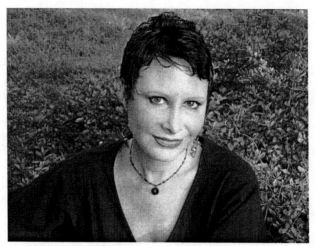

Author-Lauren Brower

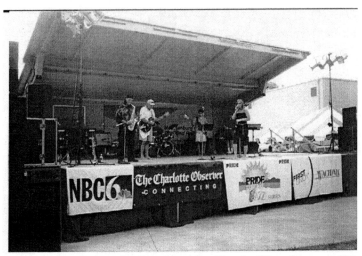

Lauren & Friends-Jazz in the Park Charlotte, NC

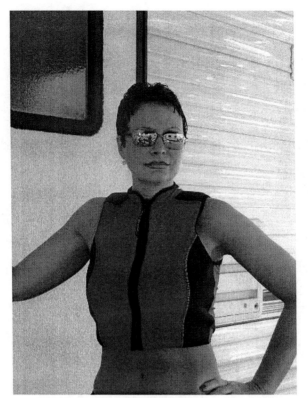

At Topsail Island-during radiation

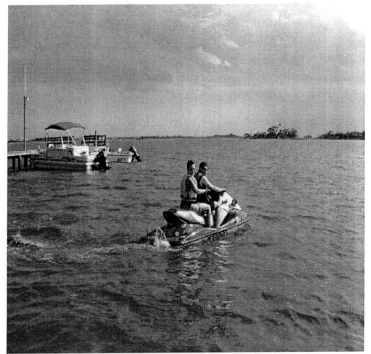

Jet Ski w/ Scott-Topsail Island

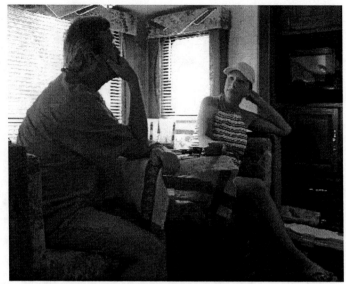

Considering the future w/ Father in Law

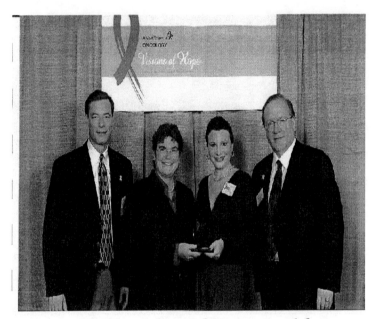

Lauren wins Visions of Hope award from
AstraZeneca

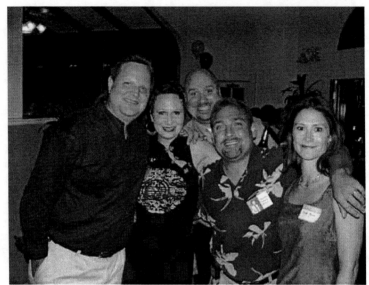

Crashing the reunion and finding old friends…
Go
SEHS

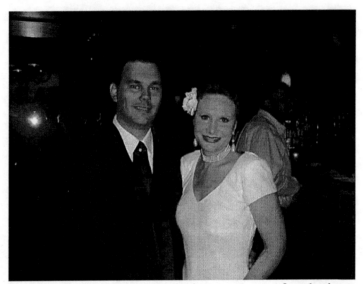

Lauren & Scott renew their vows at a fundraiser.
October 2003

Resources:

It was my desire to include some resources that had been helpful either personally or had been recommended by others that I have known through experience. There is such a wealth and myriad of information out there that locating them can be daunting and confusing. The following are books, websites and resources that I have used or were referred to me through my personal network. I have chosen not to list some of the most common, as they are fairly easy to locate and while very helpful, might not be as specific. That in no way means that I did not take advantage of them, I am simply trying to expand some of the boundaries. I also wished to include some resources specific to survivors with metastasis. Some are not even directly related to cancer but survivorship of life in general. I hope you are able to find some of them of assistance and remember none of the information provided here is intended to substitute for sound medical advice.

Books/Ebooks
(Most available at Amazon.com unless otherwise indicated.)

Don't Let the Cat Get Your Wig-Lauren Brower
(Available at Amazon.com or www.laurenandfriends.com)

I still buy green bananas-Y-ME National Breast Cancer Organization Ebook in PDF format- http://www.y-me.org/information/chestwall_local_recurrance.php
(A good source of information on recurrence)

Hope Lives! The After Breast Cancer Treatment Survival Handbook- Margit Esser Porter
(h. i. c. publishing - Advice and voices of survivors)

I'd rather Laugh - Linda Richman
(Sage advice from the coffee talk lady)

If you Could Hear What I See – Kathy Buckley
(Inspirational/humorous book and good friend)

Angel Second Class – Kathy Sumner
(Jarret Press- North Carolina Hospice Nurse)

Interruptions – Poignant Poems by the Live Poets Society of Charlotte
(Made possible by the Arts & Science Council and the Buddy Kemp Caring House-see link under support)

Advanced Breast Cancer: A Guide to Living with Metastatic Disease – Musa Mayer

Support/Advocacy

Young Survival Coalition www.youngsurvival.org

Friends…You Can Count On www.earlier.org

Buddy Kemp Caring House - Charlotte, NC www.presbyterian.org/health_services/cancer_center/support_s ervices/buddy_kemp_caring_house/

Internet

www.webmd.com

www.thewellnesscommunity.org

Specific info on metastatic disease –
www.breastcancer.org/rcr_metas_idx.html

Magazines

Mamm
www.mamm.com

Cure (Free for a limited time to survivors)
www.curetoday.com

Coping with Cancer
www.copingmag.com

These are just a smattering of the resources available and the ones that I have taken advantage of. Again I wanted to make suggestions off the beaten path. I encourage the use of the internet and library for additional info but remind everyone to never make decisions without consulting their primary caregiver and loved ones first.

Wishing you good health...

Lauren Brower